My
Kimchi
Log

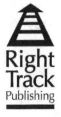

Right Track Publishing

Olathe, KS

The Fervent Fermenter is *not* a series of How-To books. It is assumed that readers are relying on instructions and recipes from other sources. These journal-style logbooks are designed for keeping records of your forays into fermenting.
Happy adventures!

My Kimchi Log
The Fervent Fermenter Series
Published by Right Track Publishing in 2017
righttrackpublishing.com

Design and Writing © 2017 Tracy Tennant
Cover kimchi image © Floriankittemann | Dreamstime.com

ISBN: 978-0-9913371-4-9

Kimchi Basics

Kimchi is a Korean dish made with fermented vegetables. It can be used in Asian-style meals, as a condiment, or eaten straight from the jar (only put it in a bowl, unless you plan on devouring it in one sitting). Kimchi is is the Korean version of sauerkraut, only spicier and with more vegetables.
It's vitamin rich with minerals, enzymes, and probiotics.

According to the Journal of Cancer Prevention, "kimchi, in general, is a healthy food recognized for its antioxidant, antiobese, cancer preventive, and other health beneficial effects." (1)

There is no single way to make kimchi; there are hundreds! The process itself (fermenting vegetables in a brine solution) is pretty straightforward, but there are hundreds of variations in regard to the kinds of vegetables and seasonings used.

Each batch can be a new flavor experience, as the final taste depends on the temperature, length of time fermenting, and the spices used to season it. That's why record-keeping is so helpful. Once you make a batch that's ooh-la-la, you will want to repeat your success over and over again.

For best results, it's recommended you follow the detailed directions from your favorite kimchi book or website. Always take proper precautions for sanitary food preparation before starting your kimchi.

1. https://www.ncbi.nlm.nih.gov/pmc/articles/PMC4285955/

You will need:

- ✓ Wide mouth quart mason jars
- ✓ Utility knife or food processor
- ✓ Kitchen pounding tool
- ✓ Large mixing bowl
- ✓ Airlock or mason lids
- ✓ Strainer
- ✓ Spoon

Ingredients to have on hand:

- Napa cabbage
- Green onions
- Daikon radish
- Garlic
- Ginger

- Ginger
- Sea salt
- Korean red pepper powder
- Sugar
- Fish sauce (optional)

Kimchi takes from 2 to 10 days to ferment, depending on desired flavor and strength. Ideal ambient temperature is 60 to 70 degrees. When the kimchi is to your liking, refrigerate it.

For instructions on making kimchi and recipes for using it, please check out the following resources!

The resources below are great go-to's for beginners:

Websites

superfoods-for-superhealth.com/kimchi-recipe.html

culturesforhealth.com/learn/natural-fermentation/how-to-ferment-vegetables/

yumuniverse.com/fermented-vegetables-make-your-own-kimchi/

Books

Ferment Your Vegetables: A Fun and Flavorful Guide to Making Your Own Pickles, Kimchi, Kraut, and More
by Amanda Feifer

The Kimchi Cookbook: 60 Traditional and Modern Ways to Make and Eat Kimchi
by Lauryn Chun and Olga Massov

Details

Vessel Size _____   # of Jars _____

Lid Type: ☐ Airlock   ☐ Other _____

Room Temp _____

Start Date ●―――――――――――●

Ingredients used: _____

_____

_____

_____

_____

Recipe retrieved from: _____

_____

☐ 2-day check / Flavor _____

☐ 4-day check / Flavor _____

☐ 7-day check / Flavor _____

Harvest Date: ●―――――――――――●

Total # fermenting days _____

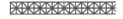

Notes:

Details

Vessel Size _____   # of Jars _____

Lid Type: ☐ Airlock   ☐ Other _____

Room Temp _____

Start Date ●_____●

Ingredients used: _____

_____

_____

_____

_____

Recipe retrieved from: _____

_____

☐ 2-day check / Flavor _____

☐ 4-day check / Flavor _____

☐ 7-day check / Flavor _____

Harvest Date: ●_____●

Total # fermenting days _____

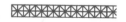 **Notes:**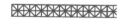

Details

Vessel Size _____   # of Jars _____

Lid Type: ☐ Airlock   ☐ Other _____

Room Temp _____

Start Date ●_____●

Ingredients used: _____

_____

_____

_____

_____

Recipe retrieved from: _____

_____

☐ 2-day check / Flavor _____

☐ 4-day check / Flavor _____

☐ 7-day check / Flavor _____

Harvest Date: ●_____●

Total # fermenting days _____

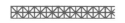 **Notes:**

Details

Vessel Size _____   # of Jars _____

Lid Type: ☐ Airlock   ☐ Other _____

Room Temp _____

Start Date ●_____●

Ingredients used: _____

_____

_____

_____

_____

Recipe retrieved from: _____

_____

☐ 2-day check / Flavor _____

☐ 4-day check / Flavor _____

☐ 7-day check / Flavor _____

Harvest Date: ●_____●

Total # fermenting days _____

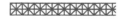 **Notes:**

Details

Vessel Size _____   # of Jars _____

Lid Type: ☐ Airlock   ☐ Other _____

Room Temp _____

Start Date ●_____●

Ingredients used: _____

_____

_____

_____

_____

Recipe retrieved from: _____

_____

☐ 2-day check / Flavor _____

☐ 4-day check / Flavor _____

☐ 7-day check / Flavor _____

Harvest Date: ●_____●

Total # fermenting days _____

Notes:

Details

Vessel Size _____   # of Jars _____

Lid Type: ☐ Airlock   ☐ Other _____

Room Temp _____

Start Date •————————————•

Ingredients used: _____

_____

_____

_____

_____

Recipe retrieved from: _____

_____

☐ 2-day check / Flavor _____

☐ 4-day check / Flavor _____

☐ 7-day check / Flavor _____

Harvest Date: •————————————•

Total # fermenting days _____

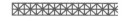

Notes:

Details

Vessel Size _____   # of Jars _____

Lid Type: ☐ Airlock   ☐ Other _____

Room Temp _____

Start Date ●_____●

Ingredients used: _____
_____
_____
_____
_____

Recipe retrieved from: _____
_____

☐ 2-day check / Flavor _____
☐ 4-day check / Flavor _____
☐ 7-day check / Flavor _____

Harvest Date: ●_____●

Total # fermenting days _____

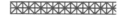

Notes:

Details

Vessel Size _____   # of Jars _____

Lid Type: ☐ Airlock   ☐ Other _____

Room Temp _____

Start Date ●_____●

Ingredients used: _____

_____

_____

_____

_____

Recipe retrieved from: _____

_____

☐ 2-day check / Flavor _____

☐ 4-day check / Flavor _____

☐ 7-day check / Flavor _____

Harvest Date: ●_____●

Total # fermenting days _____

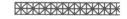

Notes:

Details

Vessel Size _____   # of Jars _____

Lid Type: ☐ Airlock   ☐ Other _____

Room Temp _____

Start Date ●————————————●

Ingredients used: _____

_____

_____

_____

_____

Recipe retrieved from: _____

_____

☐ 2-day check / Flavor _____

☐ 4-day check / Flavor _____

☐ 7-day check / Flavor _____

Harvest Date: ●————————————●

Total # fermenting days _____

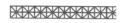 **Notes:**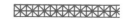

Details

Vessel Size _____   # of Jars _____

Lid Type: ☐ Airlock   ☐ Other _____

Room Temp _____

Start Date _____

Ingredients used: _____

_____

_____

_____

_____

Recipe retrieved from: _____

_____

☐ 2-day check / Flavor _____

☐ 4-day check / Flavor _____

☐ 7-day check / Flavor _____

Harvest Date: _____

Total # fermenting days _____

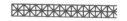 # Notes: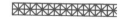

Details

Vessel Size _____   # of Jars _____

Lid Type: ☐ Airlock   ☐ Other _____

Room Temp _____

Start Date _____

Ingredients used: _____

_____

_____

_____

_____

Recipe retrieved from: _____

_____

☐ 2-day check / Flavor _____

☐ 4-day check / Flavor _____

☐ 7-day check / Flavor _____

Harvest Date: _____

Total # fermenting days _____

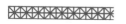 **Notes:**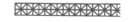

Details

Vessel Size _____   # of Jars _____

Lid Type: ☐ Airlock   ☐ Other _____

Room Temp _____

Start Date ●————————————●

Ingredients used: _____

_____

_____

_____

_____

Recipe retrieved from: _____

_____

☐ 2-day check / Flavor _____

☐ 4-day check / Flavor _____

☐ 7-day check / Flavor _____

Harvest Date: ●————————————●

Total # fermenting days _____

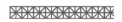 **Notes:**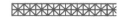

Details

Vessel Size _____   # of Jars _____

Lid Type: ☐ Airlock   ☐ Other _____

Room Temp _____

Start Date ●_____●

Ingredients used: _____

_____

_____

_____

_____

Recipe retrieved from: _____

_____

☐ 2-day check / Flavor _____

☐ 4-day check / Flavor _____

☐ 7-day check / Flavor _____

Harvest Date: ●_____●

Total # fermenting days _____

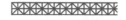 **Notes:**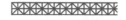

Details

Vessel Size _____   # of Jars _____

Lid Type: ☐ Airlock   ☐ Other _____

Room Temp _____

Start Date _____

Ingredients used: _____

_____

_____

_____

_____

Recipe retrieved from: _____

_____

☐ 2-day check / Flavor _____

☐ 4-day check / Flavor _____

☐ 7-day check / Flavor _____

Harvest Date: _____

Total # fermenting days _____

Notes:

Details

Vessel Size _____   # of Jars _____

Lid Type: ☐ Airlock   ☐ Other _____

Room Temp _____

Start Date ●————————————●

Ingredients used: _____
_____
_____
_____
_____

Recipe retrieved from: _____
_____

☐ 2-day check / Flavor _____

☐ 4-day check / Flavor _____

☐ 7-day check / Flavor _____

Harvest Date: ●————————————●

Total # fermenting days _____

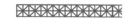 **Notes:**

Details

Vessel Size _____   # of Jars _____

Lid Type: ☐ Airlock   ☐ Other _____

Room Temp _____

Start Date ●━━━━━━━━━●

Ingredients used: _____

_____

_____

_____

_____

Recipe retrieved from: _____

_____

☐ 2-day check / Flavor _____

☐ 4-day check / Flavor _____

☐ 7-day check / Flavor _____

Harvest Date: ●━━━━━━━━━●

Total # fermenting days _____

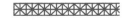

Notes:

Details

Vessel Size _____   # of Jars _____

Lid Type: ☐ Airlock   ☐ Other _____

Room Temp _____

Start Date ●_____●

Ingredients used: _____

_____

_____

_____

_____

Recipe retrieved from: _____

_____

☐ 2-day check / Flavor _____

☐ 4-day check / Flavor _____

☐ 7-day check / Flavor _____

Harvest Date: ●_____●

Total # fermenting days _____

Notes:

Details

Vessel Size _____   # of Jars _____

Lid Type: ☐ Airlock   ☐ Other _____

Room Temp _____

Start Date ●_____●

Ingredients used: _____

_____

_____

_____

_____

Recipe retrieved from: _____

_____

☐ 2-day check / Flavor _____

☐ 4-day check / Flavor _____

☐ 7-day check / Flavor _____

Harvest Date: ●_____●

Total # fermenting days _____

Notes:

Details

Vessel Size _____   # of Jars _____

Lid Type: ☐ Airlock   ☐ Other _____

Room Temp _____

Start Date ●_____●

Ingredients used: _____

_____

_____

_____

_____

Recipe retrieved from: _____

_____

☐ 2-day check / Flavor _____

☐ 4-day check / Flavor _____

☐ 7-day check / Flavor _____

Harvest Date: ●_____●

Total # fermenting days _____

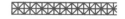 **Notes:**

Details

Vessel Size _____   # of Jars _____

Lid Type: ☐ Airlock   ☐ Other _____

Room Temp _____

Start Date ●━━━━━━━━━━━━━━●

Ingredients used: _____

_____

_____

_____

_____

Recipe retrieved from: _____

_____

☐ 2-day check / Flavor _____

☐ 4-day check / Flavor _____

☐ 7-day check / Flavor _____

Harvest Date: ●━━━━━━━━━━━●

Total # fermenting days _____

Notes:

Details

Vessel Size _____   # of Jars _____

Lid Type: ☐ Airlock   ☐ Other _____

Room Temp _____

Start Date ●——————————————●

Ingredients used: _____

_____

_____

_____

_____

Recipe retrieved from: _____

_____

☐ 2-day check / Flavor _____

☐ 4-day check / Flavor _____

☐ 7-day check / Flavor _____

Harvest Date: ●——————————————●

Total # fermenting days _____

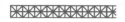 **Notes:**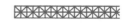

Details

Vessel Size _____   # of Jars _____

Lid Type: ☐ Airlock   ☐ Other _____

Room Temp _____

Start Date ●_____●

Ingredients used: _____

_____

_____

_____

_____

Recipe retrieved from: _____

_____

☐ 2-day check / Flavor _____

☐ 4-day check / Flavor _____

☐ 7-day check / Flavor _____

Harvest Date: ●_____●

Total # fermenting days _____

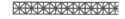 **Notes:**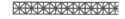

Details

Vessel Size _____   # of Jars _____

Lid Type: ☐ Airlock   ☐ Other _____

Room Temp _____

Start Date ●_____●

Ingredients used: _____

_____

_____

_____

_____

Recipe retrieved from: _____

_____

☐ 2-day check / Flavor _____

☐ 4-day check / Flavor _____

☐ 7-day check / Flavor _____

Harvest Date: ●_____●

Total # fermenting days _____

Notes:

Details

Vessel Size _____   # of Jars _____

Lid Type: ☐ Airlock   ☐ Other _____

Room Temp _____

Start Date ●_____●

Ingredients used: _____
_____
_____
_____
_____

Recipe retrieved from: _____
_____

☐ 2-day check / Flavor _____

☐ 4-day check / Flavor _____

☐ 7-day check / Flavor _____

Harvest Date: ●_____●

Total # fermenting days _____

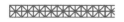 **Notes:**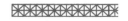

Details

Vessel Size _____   # of Jars _____

Lid Type: ☐ Airlock   ☐ Other _____

Room Temp _____

Start Date ●_____●

Ingredients used: _____

_____

_____

_____

_____

Recipe retrieved from: _____

_____

☐ 2-day check / Flavor _____

☐ 4-day check / Flavor _____

☐ 7-day check / Flavor _____

Harvest Date: ●_____●

Total # fermenting days _____

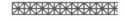

Notes:

Details

Vessel Size _____   # of Jars _____

Lid Type: ☐ Airlock   ☐ Other _____

Room Temp _____

Start Date ●_____●

Ingredients used: _____

_____

_____

_____

_____

Recipe retrieved from: _____

_____

☐ 2-day check / Flavor _____

☐ 4-day check / Flavor _____

☐ 7-day check / Flavor _____

Harvest Date: ●_____●

Total # fermenting days _____

Notes:

Details

Vessel Size _____   # of Jars _____

Lid Type: ☐ Airlock   ☐ Other _____

Room Temp _____

Start Date •_____•

Ingredients used: _____
_____
_____
_____
_____

Recipe retrieved from: _____
_____

☐ 2-day check / Flavor _____

☐ 4-day check / Flavor _____

☐ 7-day check / Flavor _____

Harvest Date: •_____•

Total # fermenting days _____

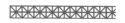 **Notes:**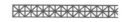

Details

Vessel Size _____   # of Jars _____

Lid Type: ☐ Airlock   ☐ Other _____

Room Temp _____

Start Date ●————————————●

Ingredients used: _____

_____

_____

_____

_____

Recipe retrieved from: _____

_____

☐ 2-day check / Flavor _____

☐ 4-day check / Flavor _____

☐ 7-day check / Flavor _____

Harvest Date: ●————————————●

Total # fermenting days _____

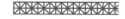 **Notes:**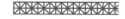

Details

Vessel Size _____   # of Jars _____

Lid Type: ☐ Airlock   ☐ Other _____

Room Temp _____

Start Date ●————————————●

Ingredients used: _____

_____

_____

_____

_____

Recipe retrieved from: _____

_____

☐ 2-day check / Flavor _____

☐ 4-day check / Flavor _____

☐ 7-day check / Flavor _____

Harvest Date: ●————————————●

Total # fermenting days _____

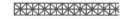

Notes:

Details

Vessel Size _____   # of Jars _____

Lid Type: ☐ Airlock   ☐ Other _____

Room Temp _____

Start Date ●_____●

Ingredients used: _____

_____

_____

_____

_____

Recipe retrieved from: _____

_____

☐ 2-day check / Flavor _____

☐ 4-day check / Flavor _____

☐ 7-day check / Flavor _____

Harvest Date: ●_____●

Total # fermenting days _____

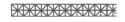 **Notes:**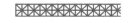

Details

Vessel Size _____   # of Jars _____

Lid Type: ☐ Airlock   ☐ Other _____

Room Temp _____

Start Date ●_____●

Ingredients used: _____

_____

_____

_____

_____

Recipe retrieved from: _____

_____

☐ 2-day check / Flavor _____

☐ 4-day check / Flavor _____

☐ 7-day check / Flavor _____

Harvest Date: ●_____●

Total # fermenting days _____

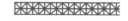

Notes:

Details

Vessel Size _____   # of Jars _____

Lid Type: ☐ Airlock   ☐ Other _____

Room Temp _____

Start Date •_____•

Ingredients used: _____

_____

_____

_____

_____

Recipe retrieved from: _____

_____

☐ 2-day check / Flavor _____

☐ 4-day check / Flavor _____

☐ 7-day check / Flavor _____

Harvest Date: •_____•

Total # fermenting days _____

Notes:

Details

Vessel Size _____   # of Jars _____

Lid Type: ☐ Airlock   ☐ Other _____

Room Temp _____

Start Date ●_____●

Ingredients used: _____

_____

_____

_____

_____

Recipe retrieved from: _____

_____

☐ 2-day check / Flavor _____

☐ 4-day check / Flavor _____

☐ 7-day check / Flavor _____

Harvest Date: ●_____●

Total # fermenting days _____

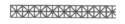 **Notes:**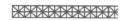

Details

Vessel Size _____   # of Jars _____

Lid Type: ☐ Airlock ☐ Other _____

Room Temp _____

Start Date ●————————————————●

Ingredients used: _____

_____

_____

_____

_____

Recipe retrieved from: _____

_____

☐ 2-day check / Flavor _____

☐ 4-day check / Flavor _____

☐ 7-day check / Flavor _____

Harvest Date: ●————————————————●

Total # fermenting days _____

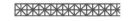

Notes:

Details

Vessel Size _____   # of Jars _____

Lid Type: ☐ Airlock   ☐ Other _____

Room Temp _____

Start Date ●―――――――――●

Ingredients used: _____
_____
_____
_____
_____

Recipe retrieved from: _____
_____

☐ 2-day check / Flavor _____
☐ 4-day check / Flavor _____
☐ 7-day check / Flavor _____

Harvest Date: ●―――――――――●

Total # fermenting days _____

Notes:

Details

Vessel Size _____   # of Jars _____

Lid Type: ☐ Airlock   ☐ Other _____

Room Temp _____

Start Date ●_____●

Ingredients used: _____

_____

_____

_____

_____

Recipe retrieved from: _____

_____

☐ 2-day check / Flavor _____

☐ 4-day check / Flavor _____

☐ 7-day check / Flavor _____

Harvest Date: ●_____●

Total # fermenting days _____

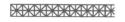 **Notes:**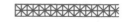

Details

Vessel Size _____   # of Jars _____

Lid Type: ☐ Airlock   ☐ Other _____

Room Temp _____

Start Date _____

Ingredients used: _____

_____

_____

_____

_____

Recipe retrieved from: _____

_____

☐ 2-day check / Flavor _____

☐ 4-day check / Flavor _____

☐ 7-day check / Flavor _____

Harvest Date: _____

Total # fermenting days _____

Notes:

Details

Vessel Size _____   # of Jars _____

Lid Type: ☐ Airlock   ☐ Other _____

Room Temp _____

Start Date ●_____●

Ingredients used: _____

_____

_____

_____

_____

Recipe retrieved from: _____

_____

☐ 2-day check / Flavor _____

☐ 4-day check / Flavor _____

☐ 7-day check / Flavor _____

Harvest Date: ●_____●

Total # fermenting days _____

Notes:

Details

Vessel Size _____   # of Jars _____

Lid Type: ☐ Airlock   ☐ Other _____

Room Temp _____

Start Date ●————————————●

Ingredients used: _____

_____

_____

_____

_____

Recipe retrieved from: _____

_____

☐ 2-day check / Flavor _____

☐ 4-day check / Flavor _____

☐ 7-day check / Flavor _____

Harvest Date: ●————————————●

Total # fermenting days _____

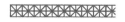 **Notes:**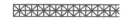

Details

Vessel Size _____   # of Jars _____

Lid Type: ☐ Airlock   ☐ Other _____

Room Temp _____

Start Date ●_____●

Ingredients used: _____
_____
_____
_____
_____

Recipe retrieved from: _____
_____

☐ 2-day check / Flavor _____

☐ 4-day check / Flavor _____

☐ 7-day check / Flavor _____

Harvest Date: ●_____●

Total # fermenting days _____

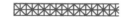

Notes:

Details

Vessel Size _____   # of Jars _____

Lid Type: ☐ Airlock   ☐ Other _____

Room Temp _____

Start Date ●————————————●

Ingredients used: _____

_____

_____

_____

_____

Recipe retrieved from: _____

_____

☐ 2-day check / Flavor _____

☐ 4-day check / Flavor _____

☐ 7-day check / Flavor _____

Harvest Date: ●————————————●

Total # fermenting days _____

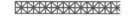

Notes:

Details

Vessel Size _____   # of Jars _____

Lid Type: ☐ Airlock   ☐ Other _____

Room Temp _____

Start Date ●_____●

Ingredients used: _____

_____

_____

_____

_____

Recipe retrieved from: _____

_____

☐ 2-day check / Flavor _____

☐ 4-day check / Flavor _____

☐ 7-day check / Flavor _____

Harvest Date: ●_____●

Total # fermenting days _____

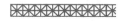 **Notes:**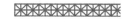

Details

Vessel Size _____   # of Jars _____

Lid Type: ☐ Airlock   ☐ Other _____

Room Temp _____

Start Date _____

Ingredients used: _____

_____

_____

_____

_____

Recipe retrieved from: _____

_____

☐ 2-day check / Flavor _____

☐ 4-day check / Flavor _____

☐ 7-day check / Flavor _____

Harvest Date: _____

Total # fermenting days _____

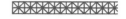# Notes:

Details

Vessel Size _____   # of Jars _____

Lid Type: ☐ Airlock   ☐ Other _____

Room Temp _____

Start Date _____

Ingredients used: _____

_____

_____

_____

_____

Recipe retrieved from: _____

_____

☐ 2-day check / Flavor _____

☐ 4-day check / Flavor _____

☐ 7-day check / Flavor _____

Harvest Date: _____

Total # fermenting days _____

Details

Vessel Size _____   # of Jars _____

Lid Type: ☐ Airlock   ☐ Other _____

Room Temp _____

Start Date _____

Ingredients used: _____

_____

_____

_____

_____

Recipe retrieved from: _____

_____

☐ 2-day check / Flavor _____

☐ 4-day check / Flavor _____

☐ 7-day check / Flavor _____

Harvest Date: _____

Total # fermenting days _____

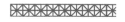 **Notes:**

Details

Vessel Size _____   # of Jars _____

Lid Type: ☐ Airlock   ☐ Other _____

Room Temp _____

Start Date •———————————•

Ingredients used: _____

_____

_____

_____

_____

Recipe retrieved from: _____

_____

☐ 2-day check / Flavor _____

☐ 4-day check / Flavor _____

☐ 7-day check / Flavor _____

Harvest Date: •———————————•

Total # fermenting days _____

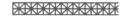 **Notes:**

Details

Vessel Size _____   # of Jars _____

Lid Type: ☐ Airlock   ☐ Other _____

Room Temp _____

Start Date ⚫_____⚫

Ingredients used: _____

_____

_____

_____

_____

Recipe retrieved from: _____

_____

☐ 2-day check / Flavor _____

☐ 4-day check / Flavor _____

☐ 7-day check / Flavor _____

Harvest Date: ⚫_____⚫

Total # fermenting days _____

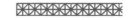 **Notes:**

Details

Vessel Size _____   # of Jars _____

Lid Type: ☐ Airlock   ☐ Other _____

Room Temp _____

Start Date ●——————————————●

Ingredients used: _____

_____

_____

_____

_____

Recipe retrieved from: _____

_____

☐ 2-day check / Flavor _____

☐ 4-day check / Flavor _____

☐ 7-day check / Flavor _____

Harvest Date: ●——————————————●

Total # fermenting days _____

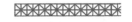 **Notes:**

Details

Vessel Size _____   # of Jars _____

Lid Type: ☐ Airlock   ☐ Other _____

Room Temp _____

Start Date ●_____●

Ingredients used: _____

_____

_____

_____

_____

Recipe retrieved from: _____

_____

☐ 2-day check / Flavor _____

☐ 4-day check / Flavor _____

☐ 7-day check / Flavor _____

Harvest Date: ●_____●

Total # fermenting days _____

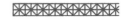 **Notes:**

Details

Vessel Size _____   # of Jars _____

Lid Type: ☐ Airlock   ☐ Other _____

Room Temp _____

Start Date ●_____●

Ingredients used: _____

_____

_____

_____

_____

Recipe retrieved from: _____

_____

☐ 2-day check / Flavor _____

☐ 4-day check / Flavor _____

☐ 7-day check / Flavor _____

Harvest Date: ●_____●

Total # fermenting days _____

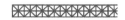 **Notes:**

CPSIA information can be obtained
at www.ICGtesting.com
Printed in the USA
LVHW010952210723
753106LV00008B/78